Dynamic Kicking for Beginners

By Master Lady L. Reed

Copyright 2023 Lady L. Reed

Printed in the United States of America

Neither the author, instructors nor the school R.A.M.A & Wellness Club LLC assumes any responsibility for injuries acquired while following directions from this book. Always consult your doctor first for your health and well-being.

Dynamic

1.   A process of constant change, activity, or progress
2.   Positive attitude and full of energy and new ideas
3.   A force that stimulates change or progress within a system or process

TABLE OF CONTENTS

DEDICATION

I dedicate this book to my husband who never ceased to encourage me, my children whom I love, my real friends, my students, and my teachers.

INTRODUCTION

My Story

Being a martial artist, I realized that for me to be able to execute my techniques stronger and more refined, I must build up my muscles. Since I've worked so hard on my flexibility, my strength is another thing that I must constantly work on.

I have female friends who are simple housewives, and I noticed their loose muscles, especially around the butt, thighs, and arms. I look at my own body and I know my core and shoulders need more exercise too.

Because I am so prone to back issues, I am continuously trying out exercises or movements that help alleviate the pain. That is how I learned that some Yoga asanas and Qigong could heal and support health.

If you see me now and all my exercises on the internet, you probably cannot ever imagine that I also had been through a lot of pain physically, mentally, and emotionally.

It is easy to choose being a victim of your past and circumstances. It is easy to blame someone or something for the diseases or uncomfortable state that you find yourself in.

I must admit that I also used to be a victim.

Just a decade and a half ago, the world seemed to be a horrible place to live in. Some people are mean, and I am being judged all the time. I was completely in need of saving. I was suffering.

Although I went through physical, emotional, and psychological trauma, I knew deep inside that I had to keep on. I searched for ways to heal myself.

I had sciatica, herniated disc, and scoliosis. I also experienced the beginning of rheumatism on the knees apart from having hyperthyroid with Basedow disease.

I read a lot of books, watched a lot of videos, and went to a lot of classes. I will not say that I'm in perfect health now nor my body is perfectly toned. But since I've been physically active, I feel that I am now in my best form at the age of 48.

Dynamic Kicking helps in keeping my legs and back strong. When I combine it with Yoga, Qigong, Weight-lifting, and other martial arts styles I practice, I can truly say that I am better each day.

MINDSET

When you set a goal, you must watch your mindset. It must be positive and uplifting that nothing can stop you in achieving your goal.

As they say, nothing positive can come out of a negative mind.

Before I started working on this book, I had to check my mindset too. I almost did not sit and finish this book. I was in doubt because I was looking out there in the world of martial arts.

There are too many books written on martial arts already. Most martial artists learned how to kick from beginning on. Yet, there are older martial artists who stopped training and can't even kick to the knee. Why is that?

Yes, it's their mindset. Sometime in their lives, they let their environment influence their mindset and stop themselves from keeping on.

I also have a DVD done called Dynamic Kicking, and I used the photograph from that video. After re-watching that video, I realized that I was so nervous when I was filming it that I couldn't talk much about what Dynamic Kicking is for.

If your intention is to defend yourself or your loved ones, then kicking is just one of the techniques that you can use in doing so.

If your intention is to be fit, you can use dynamic kicking to lose weight and build up your legs and cardio.

If your intention is to be a better athlete and be able to compete and win in tournaments, you can use dynamic kicking too and have the mind of a champion.

Never give up.

"The most beautiful experience we can have is the mysterious. It is the fundamental emotion which stands at the cradle of true art and science. Whoever does not know it and can no longer marvel, is as good as dead, and his eyes are dimmed." – Albert Einstein

EXERCISE

Regardless of your goal, exercise is important to do. The secret is in the repetition and how you feel about it.

You can take my words and apply it to other areas of your life. You will see that even in trying to be successful, it's all about mindset and the number of times you exercise your skills.

When you exercise, you must do it with a positive feeling. You can try it with a frown, and you will find the movement difficult. When you try it with a smile, any movement will be easy.

It is medically suggested to ask your physician first before you do any kind of exercise or before you follow what I'll be teaching here.

Most of them would say, at least 30 minutes of physical activity daily is needed to keep up your health, lower your metabolic risks, lose weight, lower your blood pressure, and improve your mood.

Before you do Dynamic Kicking, you must warm up. I prefer doing Cross-Tapping after doing a set of Jumping Jacks. You can start by tapping your knees for 30 seconds. Later, you can do it longer, like 1-3 minutes.

The late Jack Lalane believed in exercises. He advised everyone to set a goal, exercise daily but don't strain, and what matters is what you do with what you have.

Remember that you must warm your muscles and tendons first.

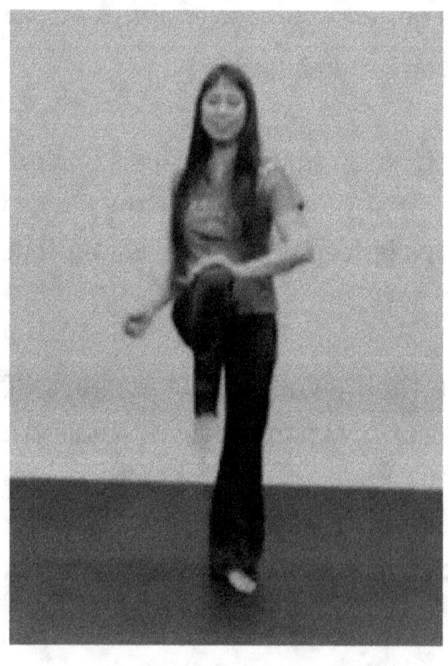

Cross-Tapping is lifting your knee as high as you can and tapping it with the opposite hand as the photo shows using left and right. You can count your taps to a hundred or simply do it for a minute. It is one of the Kinesiology exercises that activates your left and right brain hemisphere.

There are other variations of cross-tapping. One is when you tap the inner-sole of your foot with the opposite hand. The second one is when you tap the outer-sole of your foot with the opposite hand. These two variations also open your hips.

After such warm-up, you can do the following series of stretching exercises in the next chapter.

"There are no truer words than those born of experience" – old Proverb

STRETCHING

As I mentioned on my DVD Dynamic Stretching, we must stretch our body as often as we can. This set of stretching exercises targets the hips, legs, and back muscles.

If you already practice yoga, you know most of them already. Just remember that when you hold the position, it is what people would call static stretching. If you continuously change position, it is what you'd call dynamic stretching.

Some static stretching though can be transformed into isometric stretching wherein you add the contraction of muscles for 30 seconds and releasing it.

For example, when you open your legs as wide as you can to do a split, you can press your feet against the ground for 30 seconds, then release it. You will notice that you can go lower to do it again.

Go as far as you can and know the feeling of being stretched and being in pain. Stretching shouldn't be a painful experience, but you should feel that stretching feeling. If you don't push a little further than you are used to, you will not get further in your flexibility.

Before you try to do a side split though, try to do a Cossack Squat and its' variations.

Cossack Squat

If you have not had knee surgery or any damage on your knees, you can stretch by doing a Cossack squat. Bend with the left first while you leave the right leg straight out to your side. Your adductor muscles would thank you for it.

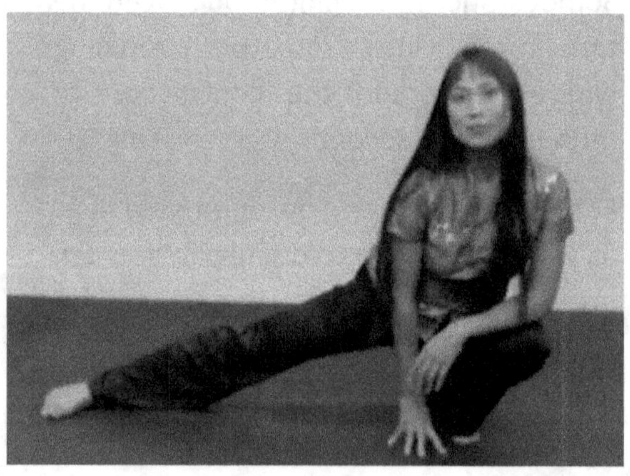

Then switch to the right side by bending the right leg and leaving the left leg straight out to your side. The feet should be parallel to each other. The back should be as straight as you can so you can also improve your balance and strength on your foot. You can also support yourself with one hand on the floor. If you have knee issue, of course, you may not be able to go lower by bending your knee.

Do this at least 10 repetitions on both sides.

Another variation is for having a high front kick. You can turn your straight leg and hips. It is best if you put your hands on the side of your legs as you bring your chest towards your knee.

Remember to keep your back straight and feel how the hamstring muscles on the back of your thigh are being stretched. Your calf muscle will also be stretched with this while you have your toes pointing upwards. Bend forward from your hips.

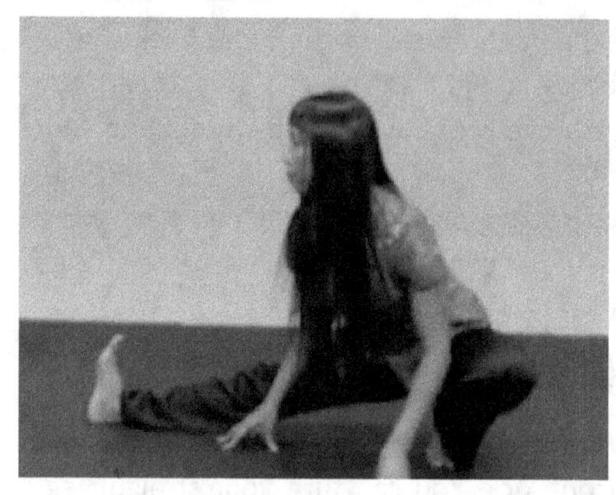
20

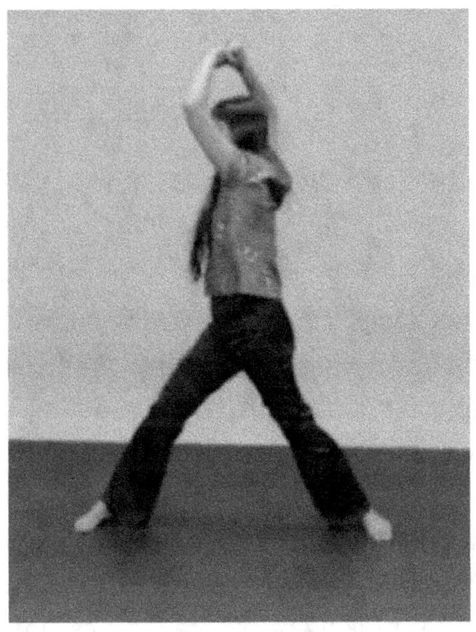

It is also important to stretch your spine. With legs wide open, you can lift your arms over your head and turn your upper body to the left and then to the right side. It will stretch your obliques and make your hips and spine flexible.

If you are having lower back pain, bending to your sides would do wonders. It stretches your quadratus lumborum muscles and your anterior serratus muscles too.

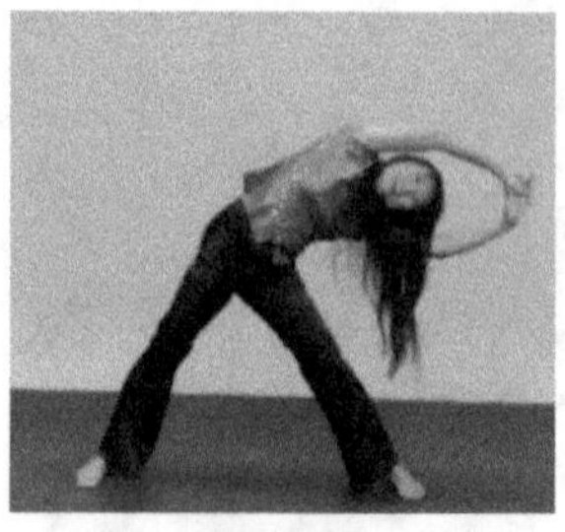

Keep your legs straight as you bend as far as you can without hurting. You can combine bending with your breathing to achieve more flexibility.

Bending backwards with your arms above your head will help you with your posture. It is like making a cobra stance in a standing position. This stretch may also help alleviate your back pain.

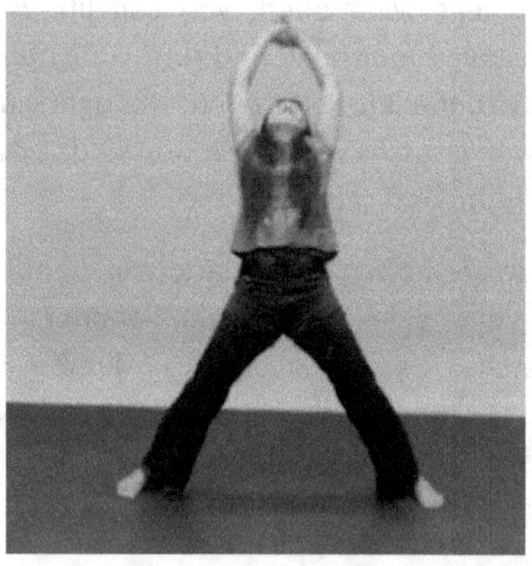

One way to stretch your hamstrings is to bend forward from your hips with straight legs. Keep your back straight as you touch the floor and stand up straight again.

If you can't touch the floor yet, bend your knees like you are doing a squat. Hold on to your feet as you make your knees straight. Do it a few times.

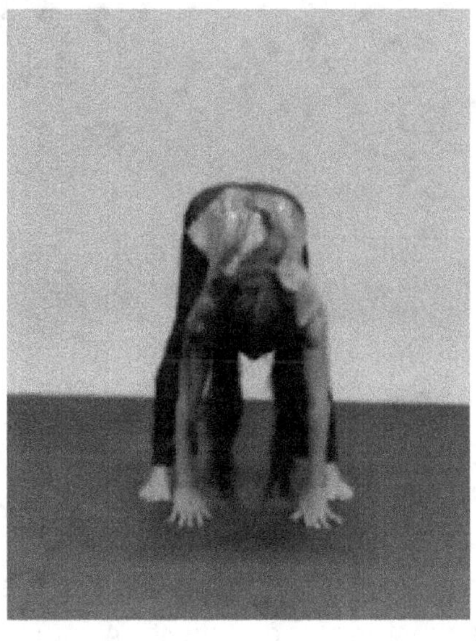

Next step after bending forward will be bringing your nose to your knee. Do this one side after the other, with legs wide apart without bending the knees.

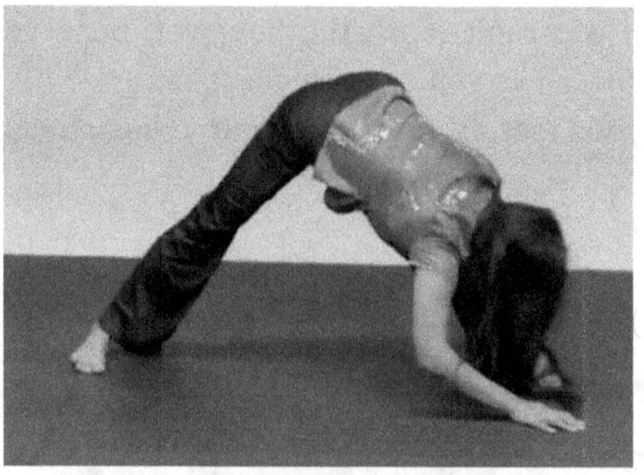

It is best to breathe out when you are leaning down and breathe in as you get up straight again.

If you go on a deep lunge, you will open your hip flexors too. Make sure you keep your back straight when you do it. I call it a "Knight Pose" in R.A.M.A. because it is like kneeling first, then adjusting your other knee on the floor further away from the other knee that is 90 degrees from the ground. When you do this, your back must be kept straight.

An ancient method of stretching is going on a horse stance or sumo stance. You can start by putting your legs wide apart and bending your knees. It is best to test the strength of your inner thigh and is almost as good as doing squats.

One last stretching is to swing your arms from left to right while keeping your legs straight at the front. It will loosen your arms, elbows, wrist, and spine. In Qigong, there are variations of this. Feel free to choose one.

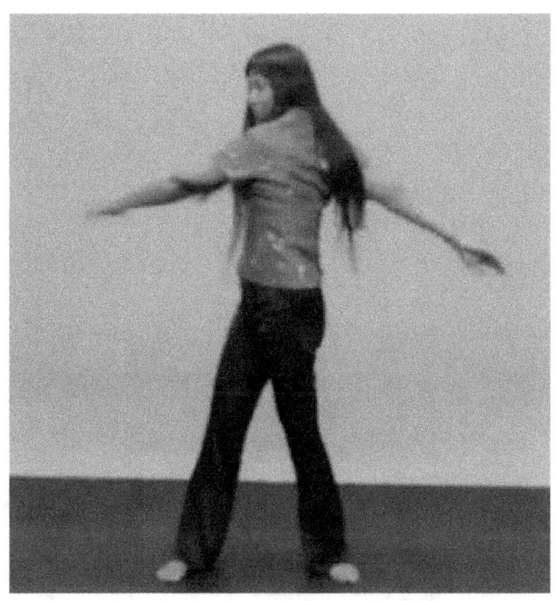

"What hurts you, blesses you. Darkness is
your candle." - Rumi

MAKING IT A HABIT

The trick to perfecting anything in life is making it a habit. If you practice the warmup exercises with stretching regularly, it will help keep you fit to do dynamic kicking or other cardiovascular activities.

Remember that it takes 21 days to keep something a habit. It's a good habit if you take care of yourself by spending time moving your body. Once you do it regularly, it will become a reflex. Your body will thank you for it.

It is in the repetition that makes you better each time. If you choose to do one kind of kick a thousand times, that one kick will matter compared to someone's who has never done any kicking.

Doing exercises with stretching together with a positive mindset will help you on your way of self-disciple and wellness. Wellness of our being is the new wealth.

DIFFERENT KICKS

If you think that a kick is just a kick, you are right. If you want to know more about the different kinds of kicks, you may read on. As you know, we all have two legs for walking, standing, running, jumping, squatting, dancing, or kicking.

Knowing the simple anatomy of your legs helps in understanding why it is important for you to build up your leg muscles. The simple knowledge that you need strong leg muscles to support your whole body is common knowledge.

Dynamic Kicking is not new at all. Everything that you will read in this book is already out there. For example, Martial artists Bill Superfoot Wallace and James Lew authored their books on dynamic kicking 30 years ago. So why am I making this book?

Just like most things in the world of martial arts, the number of female martial artists are low compared to males. Therefore, this will be the first book on dynamic kicking done by a female martial artist who is trained in multiple styles of martial arts that shows the kicking technique using bar codes.

Like my other book Shibashi Qigong Fountain of Wellness, I used bar codes as link to short instructional videos that you could easily follow. Simply scan the code with the use of Google Search bar and click the link. Please feel free to subscribe to my Youtube Channel and follow me on Social Media platforms.

There are different kinds of kicks. Each kick can be done with spinning, hopping, and jumping. What will be listed here are the basic standing kicks.

In most kicks, you will have to start with a fighting stance. In a fighting stance, your heels should be perpendicular to each other wherein the other foot toes are pointing diagonally outward while having your hands up.

Fighting stances look different from others because it depends on what style of martial arts you practice or who is your instructor.

For beginners, it doesn't matter much if you just follow along. A kick is a kick, and we all have two legs. There is nothing that you can do wrong with kicking.

Work on your balance, flexibility, strength, endurance, timing, speed, and distance.

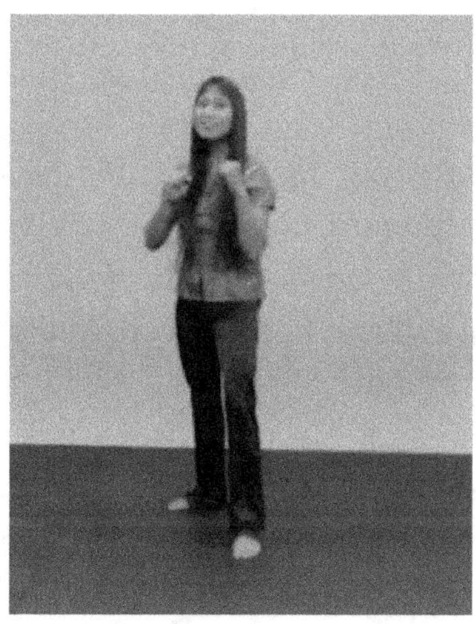

Balance is important so you can stand on one leg as you kick.

Flexibility for the height of your kick.

Strength to knock out someone with your kick or break a bone with it.

Endurance is for you to keep on kicking.

Timing is for you to know when to attack or counter.

Speed is for you to be faster than your opponent.

Distance is for kicking. If the opponent closes on you, make sure that your hand techniques are just as good defense.

FRONT STRETCH KICK

Start with your fighting stance having your left leg forward, then just swing your right leg straight up in front of you without bending it. Keep both legs straight as you do the movement.

Other styles of Martial arts have their arms on the side of their body when they kick. I prefer to have my elbows close to my ribs and my fist close to my face for protection.

When you throw that front stretch kick, make your aim as high as if you are going to kick someone who is standing behind you. Poke his/her eyes with your toes. It is as effective as a scorpion kick that requires great flexibility.

Front Kick

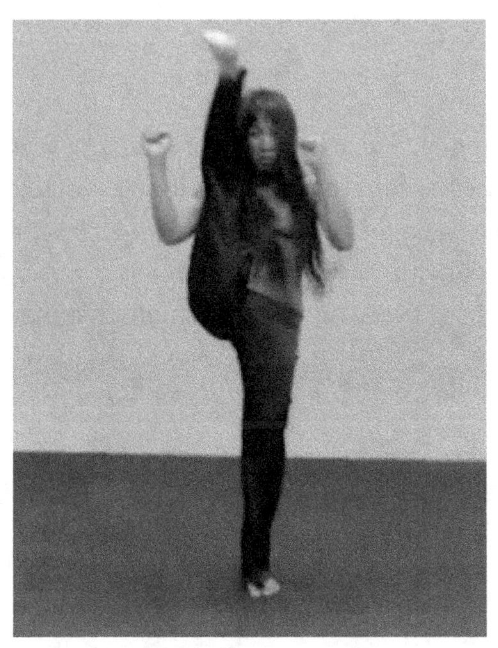

When you do a front thrust kick, you will have to lift your knee first before you extend your kick. Watch out how you kick with the ball of your foot. Pull your toes towards your body to avoid breaking them upon impact.

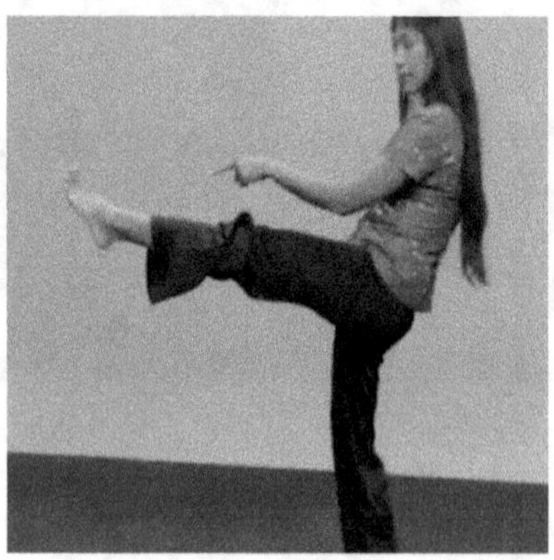

When you extend it, use your hip to push it. This kick is ideal for opening doors, or for stopping someone rushing into you.

You can kick to the knee, to the solar flexus or straight up to the throat.

Front Thrust Kick ✏️

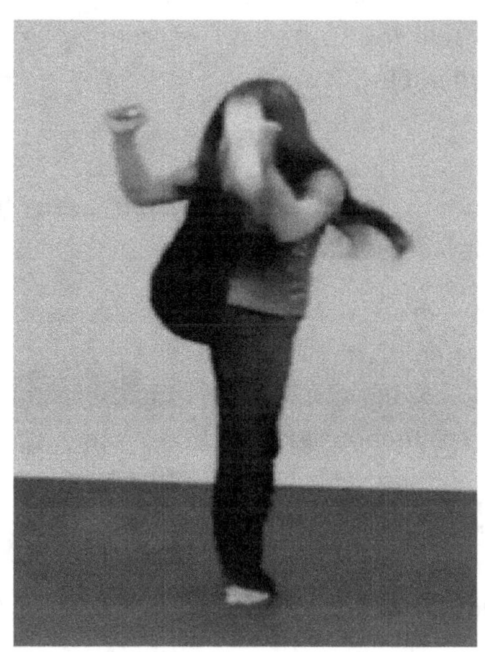

This is the first kick that is used in most fighting situations. You'll find it being used in Kickboxing, Muay Thai and Kungfu.

If you use it in combination, it will be like throwing two punches first, then front thrust kick. Or with left leg forward, do a left-hand back fist, follow it with a left punch, then front thrust kick to the stomach.

These combinations are common when you are sparring in a class or competing in a tournament.

Common kicking combination with front trust kick would be:

a)   front thrust kick, alternate leg roundhouse kick
b)   front thrust kick with the front leg, then roundhouse kick with the same leg
c)   front thrust kick with the front leg, then sidekick with the same leg
d)   front thrust kick with the rear leg, followed by a spinning back kick.

A sidekick is a common kick that is perfected in films by Bruce Lee and Chuck Norris.

You must raise your knee in front of you and as you do that movement, you will have to pivot the other leg that you are standing on. Then kick out straight on your side while keeping the position of your foot horizontal to the floor.

You can do it easier and get more power into it if you step behind first before kicking out.

This sidekick can also be done in 3 levels: to the knee, to the ribcage and to the throat or the face. If you are going to use it for self-defense, remember to kick to the knee. It will stop your opponent. Depending on how strong you kick, you can bust that person's knee and the fight is over.

All sidekicks must be in a straight line wherein your toes, knees, hips, and shoulders are in one line.

Sidekick

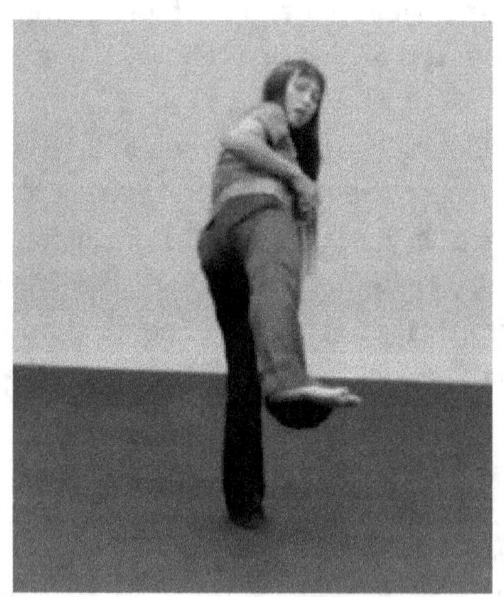

38

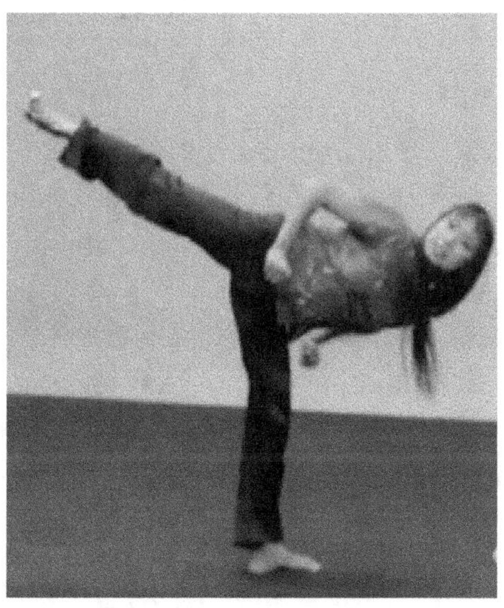

A sidekick is also prominent in Jeetkunedo. It is like the straight lead of the lower limbs.

You can combine it with hopping, jumping, and spinning. And it looks great on films if you do it very high.

If you see someone demonstrating how to they can kick straight up to the ceiling with a sidekick, be impressed. They are either born flexible or they worked hard on their flexibility. It is just a demonstration of their flexibility, not necessarily their strength. Besides, what are they kicking up the ceiling?

This kick is executed like a sidekick, but knee just comes straight up on your side. Then the kick is only from the lower leg coming from the back.

If you are standing on your left leg, you will have to lift your right leg up on the side as you pivot the left. The position of the foot is just as important. It should look like you are slapping someone's face with the top of your foot.

In some styles though, they'd use the ball of their foot when they do a roundhouse kick. In either way, it is right.

You can use a roundhouse kick in 3 levels like a sidekick: a kick to the knee, a kick to the ribcage, a kick to the side of the head.

Some people kick straight up to the ceiling for demonstration of their flexibility as well.

Roundhouse Kick

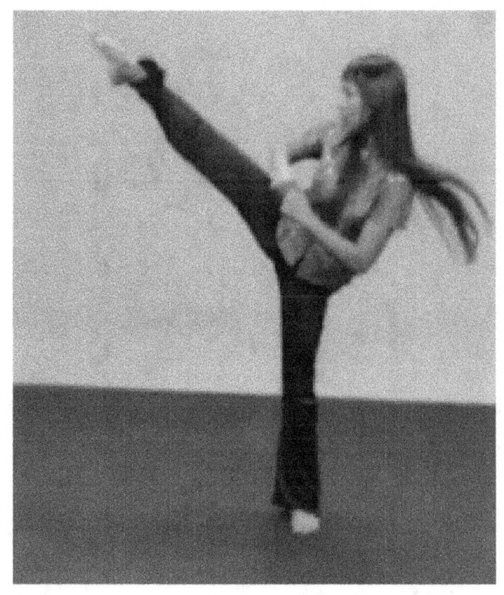

This is my favorite kick. Grandmaster Leo Fong gave me the nickname "Nutcracker" for it when he watched me spar. Then Grandmaster David L. Reed told him stories of me kicking several martial artists in the nuts.

I call the act of executing an effective front snap kick "Ring the Bell". It is the number one technique for women's self-defense.

Front Snap Kick

Always be careful in practicing the front snap kick. Some people who haven't been exercising for a long time tend to pull or tear a muscle easily.

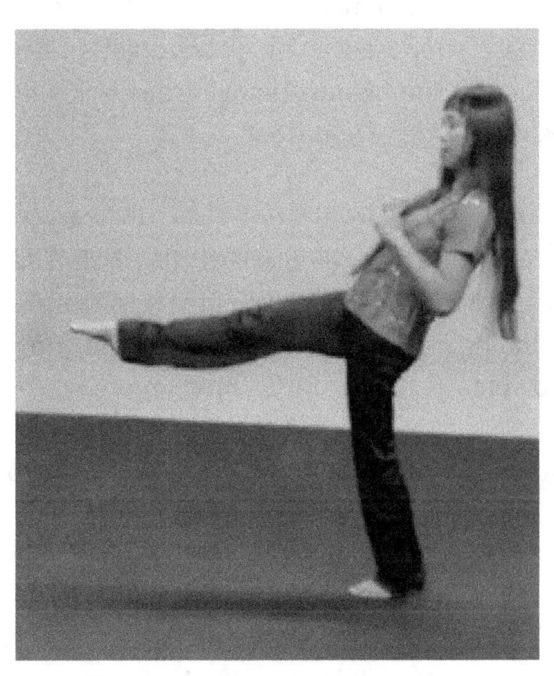

Like its name, you simply swing your leg in a circular motion from inside going outside. You are supposed to hit your target's head or face at the highest point of this kick with the outer side of your foot.

It can be a devastating kick if you hit someone on the temple with this kick. Like most kicks, you can execute this from a stranding position, or add it into your jump and spin.

It can be used in a combination of kicks to intimidate your opponent.
Like the roundhouse kick and sidekick, this crescent kick looks good in films.

Because of its impressive circular movement, Kungfu has it too. When they execute it, they demonstrate it by hitting their hand with that kick.

Inside-Out Crescer ✏️

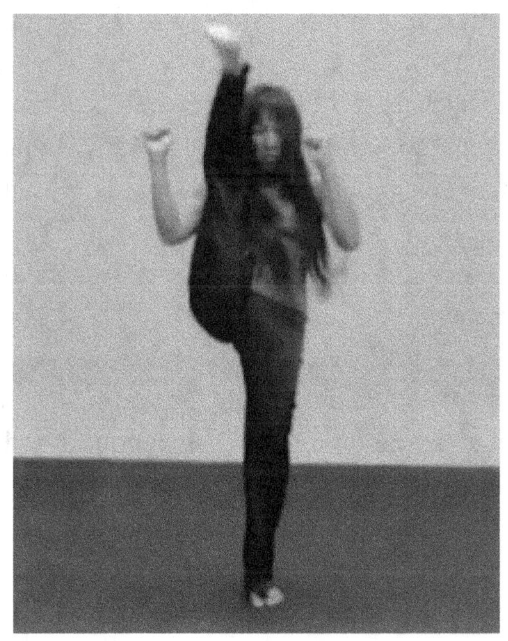

This is the opposite direction of the inside outside crescent kick. Also called as Axe kick.

You can start again with your fighting stance having the left leg in front. Swing your right leg going in circular motion going from the outside, lifting the straight right leg up in front. Then simply pull down your leg like an axe. Your heel should hit the back of the head of your opponent.

This kick is a finishing kick. It is ideal for kicking someone who is already bending down after you pull the opponent.

You would need timing to act fast in using this kick.

Like the Outside Inside Crescent kick, you can practice this with using your hand as your target.

Outside-In Crescer ✏️

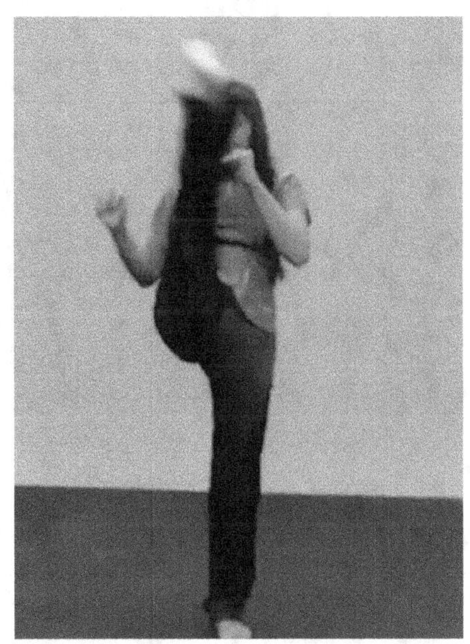

Like the name says, a back kick is for kicking someone behind you. Since we don't have eyes behind our head, it is very important to look over our shoulders before we kick to ensure hitting the target.

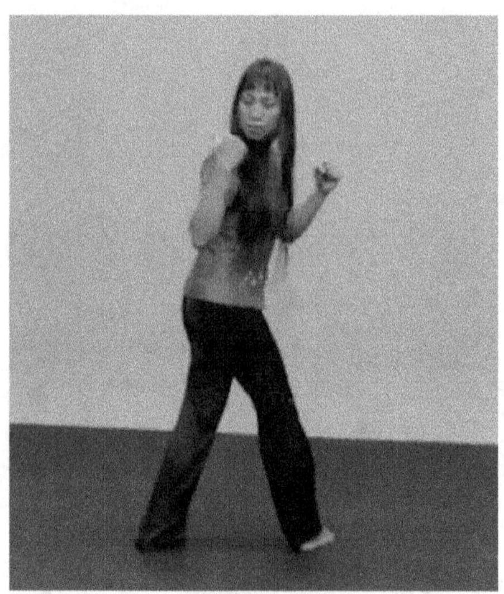

Back kick can be a strong kick like those of a horse/mule, that's why some styles call it also a mule kick.

If you are standing on your left leg, you'll have to bend forward at the same time you bend your right leg and look over your right shoulder, then extend that bent leg into a kick. Your toes should be pointing down and you should be kicking with the heel of your foot.

You can use a back kick to someone rushing towards you from behind or combine it with spinning as a defense against a roundhouse kick of your opponent.

Advance levels of martial artists combine the back kick with spinning and jumping.

If you watch old videos of Benny "The Jet" Urquidez, and Don "The Dragon" Wilson, you will see how effective back kicks are.

Practice your speed on executing a back kick.

Work on your glutes and hamstrings to gain more power for this kick.

If you are slow and you know it, just choose not to use it. You could be jammed by your opponent while you are spinning slow.

Back Kick

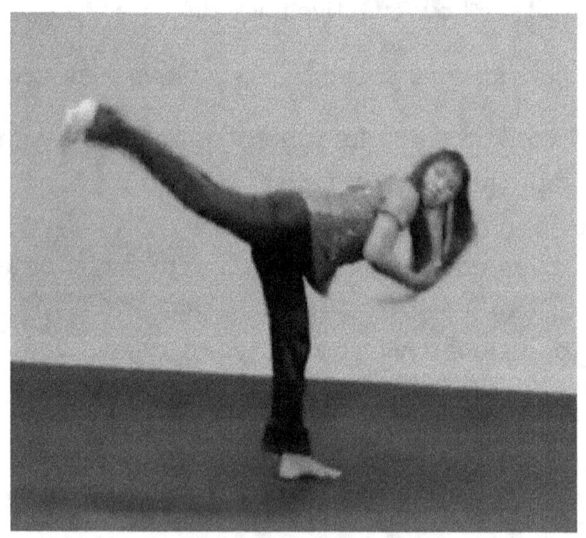

Like most of the kicking techniques, you must stretch for you the able to bring your leg up. If your sartorius and gracilis muscles are not stretched, you will not be able to kick higher for the oblique kick which will be a good, surprising kick to the face of anyone attacking you from the front.

You can execute this kick lower too. If done so, you will recognize it as one of the Wing Chun and Jeet Kune Do kicks as well. It is called a stomp kick for other styles. Doesn't it make sense?

It is used as an intercepting kick against any front kick coming from the front leg of your opponent, or simply stomping at your opponent's knees to dislocate it.

Yet it is considered a deceiving kick. If you can execute an oblique kick fast and high enough, the result can be a knockout.

Most Taekowndo practitioners combines this with a low roundhouse kick and therefore can be deceiving.

Oblique

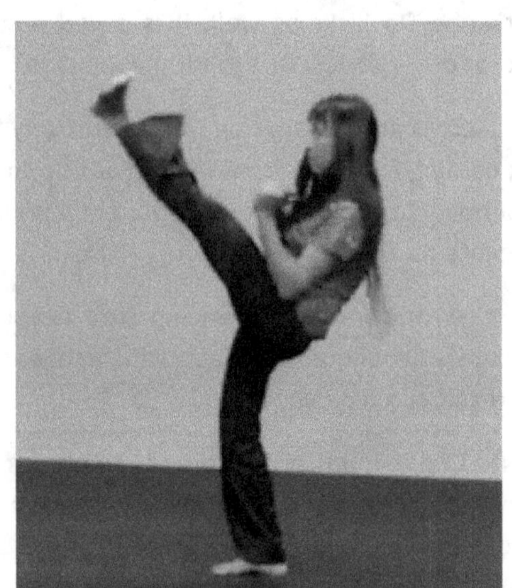

Our knees are pretty strong. It is like our elbows. It can be hurtful to someone or to yourself. The only way to condition it is by bracing yourself for the impact.

As you know, a knee is a hinge joint covered by patella. Thus, there is no muscle to build other than your hip flexors and quads.

When you kick someone with your knee, make sure you have a good balance and point down your toes.

If you watch action films, you'll see this kind of kick often. You can knee kick someone on the stomach, and on the face.

You can use it in a self-defense technique. I think Krav Maga made it also visible on videos wherein you can use it in a choking situation. When choked and pushed on a wall, you break the choker's arm with an inward-downward block/strike, elbow the face, grab the back of the neck, and pull it down to your knee strike.

If you are a Tang Soo Do practitioner, you would notice that only the Chil Sung Forms include the knee kick. Chil Sung E Roh Hyung and Chil Sung O Roh Hyung have it. It is hidden in the Naihanji Forms too.

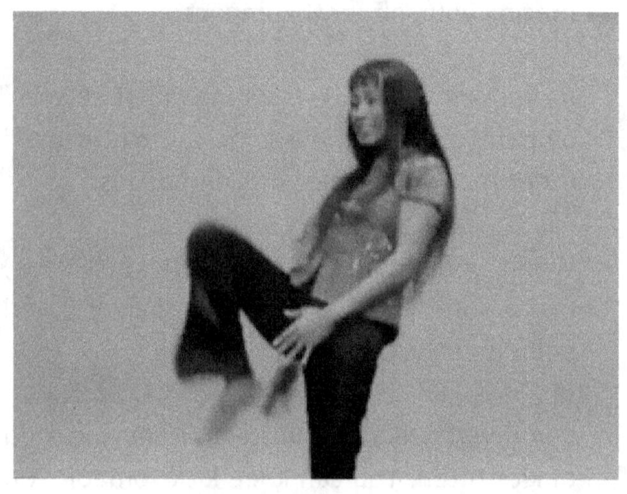

Knee Kick

Sweeping someone can be considered unfair, but it is effective if done fast and unpredictable.

I was swept by a Tang Soo Do Grandmaster when I sparred him. I was just a red belt then when we sparred. I was able to punch him in the head, which was disrespectful from me. He swept me in retaliation, and I landed on my face.

To execute a sweep though, you would have to squat down and then throw your other leg in a circular motion on the floor wherein it would hit the other person's ankle.

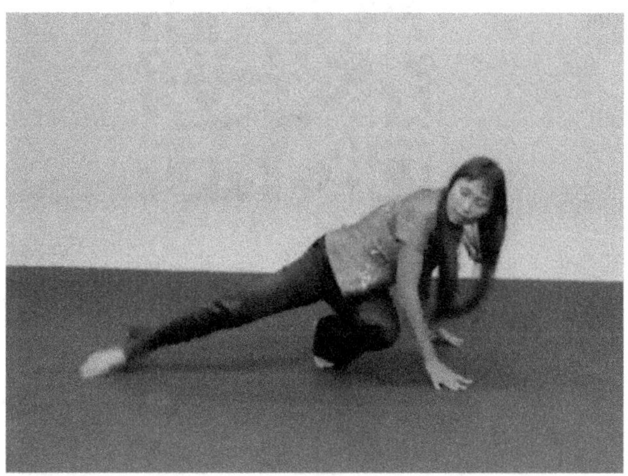

Another way would be just like hooking the other person's leg with your leg, using your heel to throw him/her off balance.

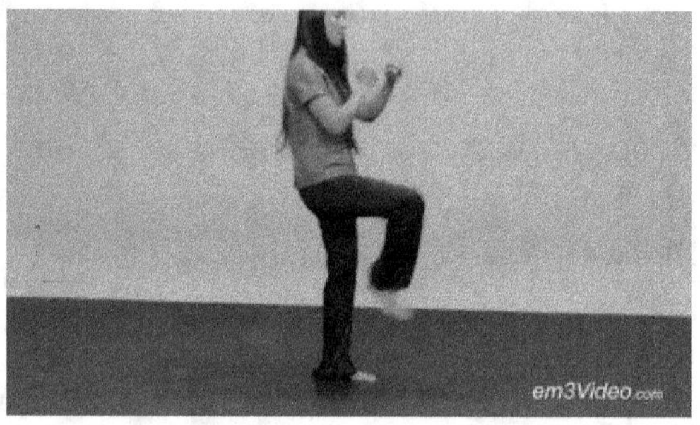

Leg Sweep

STOMP KICK

A stomp kick is from the word stomping. Yes, it is stomping on someone's knee as a kick for self-defense. It is a variation of the oblique kick.

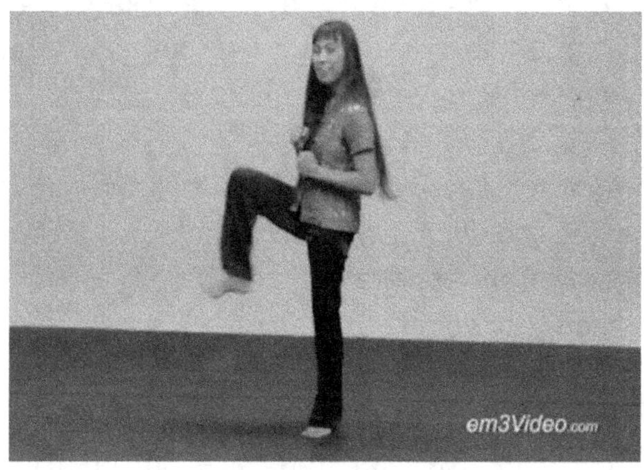

Stomp Kick

A hook kick is one of the advanced kicks. You'll need good balance, flexibility, strength in the legs, and coordination.

Stand on your left leg, do a high sidekick 45 degrees to front and then pull the heel across the opponent's temple.

Another way is to spin first, look over your right shoulder, do a high sidekick 6 inches away from your target's head and hook his head with your heel.

Most martial artists use a spinning hook kick for demonstration too, like in breaking boards. They combine it with a roundhouse kick.

Like all the other kicks, one can also add a jump to this kick to make it look like gymnastics or dance.

You need timing too to execute this devastating kick to knock someone out.

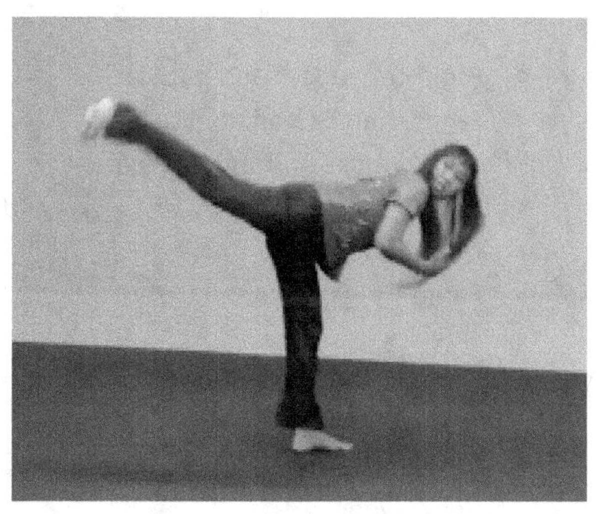

MY FAVORITE KICKING COMBINATIONS

- Front thrust kick and back kick
- Front snap kick and oblique kick
- Roundhouse and spinning back kick
- Same leg front thrust kick and roundhouse kick
- Same leg roundhouse kick and sidekick
- Outside-Inside Crescent kick and Inside-Outside Crescent Kick
- Outside-Inside Crescent kick and a floor sweep
- Roundhouse and spinning hook kick
- Low and high roundhouse kick
- Low and high sidekick

Once you have mastered all the kicking techniques standing, you can start adding it to hopping, jumping, and more spinning.

IRON LEGS

Many claimed to be masters of iron hands, but hardly anyone claimed to be masters of iron legs. Many would also say that they need a true teacher to achieve such a level of state. In any case, one must be determined to diligently practice, endure the difficulty of practicing, and be patient with oneself.

Practicing dynamic kicking will improve your flexibility, endurance, and speed for sure. You can start kicking on bags to get more power on your legs. Before kicking though, you may use a liniment or dit da jow to keep your legs from getting injured.

The use of liniment or dit da jow has been ingrained in the traditional martial arts. Always wash your hands after applying it on your body parts. Avoid touching your eyes with it on your hands.

Remember to use that Chinese herb so that the risk of internal hemorrhage will be prevented. Also be aware of your breath when you kick and how you execute your movement.

Kicking bags is a form of conditioning. In the old days, karate practitioners used to kick each other. Some shaolin monks used to get hit on their legs as well. You would lessen the risk of being injured when someone kicked you or you kick someone's conditioned leg if you have conditioned legs yourself. It happened to some fighters before, and it can be seen on Muy Thai or Kickboxing fights.

If you happen to injure your ankle or knee like a sprain or pulled muscle, the first aid would be to do R.I.C.E. Rest it, ice it, compress it, and elevate it.

ACKNOWLEDGEMENTS

I would thank my first Taekwondo instructor if I could remember his name. I can't, so I would have to give it to my own Grandmaster David L Reed who taught all the Tang Soo Do kicks I needed to be good in martial arts and Grandmaster Darryl Khalid for accepting us in the Universal Tang Soo Do Alliance.

I would also give thanks to Grandmaster Leo Fong, who passed away on Feb. 18, 2022, for all the wisdom and knowledge he passed to us in Reed's Active Martial Arts & Wellness Club. Thanks to Dr. Z for improving my Jeet Kune Do skill.

A special thanks to Sifu Greg Yau as well for demonstrating the power of Wing Chun kicks.

Thanks to GM Don Warrener and GM Val Mijalovic for the photography and DVD of Dynamic Kicking.

"The greatest warriors are those who are the greatest healers." - Musashi

ABOUT THE AUTHOR

The author, Lady L Reed is a native of Manila, Philippines. She migrated to USA at the age of 38 with her children after getting married to her American husband. She lived in Germany for almost 20 years and is fluent in German language as well as English. Her mother tongue is Tagalog.

She is a graduate of Stiftung Grone Schule in Hamburg, Germany as Certified Office Clerk, finished "Heilpraktiker" course in Institut fuer Berufliche Weiterbildung, a Certified Massage Therapist in A2Z School in Los Angeles, and an ordained minister of MSIA Church.

She started in martial arts at the age of 16. Her won 2nd place on her first Tang Soo Do tournament in Tucson, Arizona in 2015, 1st place in United States Hall of Fame Tournament in 2016, Grand champion in Shinjimasu Open Tournament in 2017, 1st place in Norco Traditional Taekwondo Tournament in 2018, Grand champion in Central Coast Tournament, Lompoc in 2019.

Since 2014, she's been training and teaching in various martial arts styles. Sifu Divina Martens, Grandmaster David L Reed, Grandmaster Leo Fong (RIP), Grandmaster Eric Lee, Grandmaster Darryl Khalid, Sifu Dr. Z, Sifu Greg Yau were her instructors.

She also attended seminars from Guro Dan Inosanto, Guro Master V, Guro Roger Agbulos, Grandmaster Thomas Caulfield, Art Camacho, Grandmaster Don Baird, Kungfu Cowboy, Vince Cecere, Soke Big Cat Frederick Peterson, Shihan Jacob Bresler, Olivier Gruner, Master Cesar Pacol, Grandmaster Robert Price, Sifu Feliz Machias, and Sifu Greglon Lee.

She also trained with Guiseppe Dmitry, Eric Gold, Master Alfred Urquidez, Grandmaster James Culpepper, Grandmaster Juerg Zigler (RIP), Jeff Jeds, Shihan Allan Woodman, Sifu Clark Tang, Sifu Wong Long Chin, Sifu Samuel Kwok, Sifu Howard Lin, Shuny Bee, Guro Manny Taningco, Grandmaster Mark Gerry, Grandmaster Philip Turner, Master Chris Wolf, Master Juan Rodriguez, Steven Lambert, and Nick Palma.

Having been inducted in several Martial Arts Hall of Fame from 2016-2023, she is known and respected in the martial arts community.

Other than martial arts, she has acted on at least 8 indie films, modeled a couple of fashion shows, and danced with singer Marie Parie and the Mojorisin Band in Hollywood from 2017-2019.

She also authored and published some books since 2019. Being an editor of R.A.M.A. News eNewsletter and learning 8 other foreign languages are some of her hobbies.

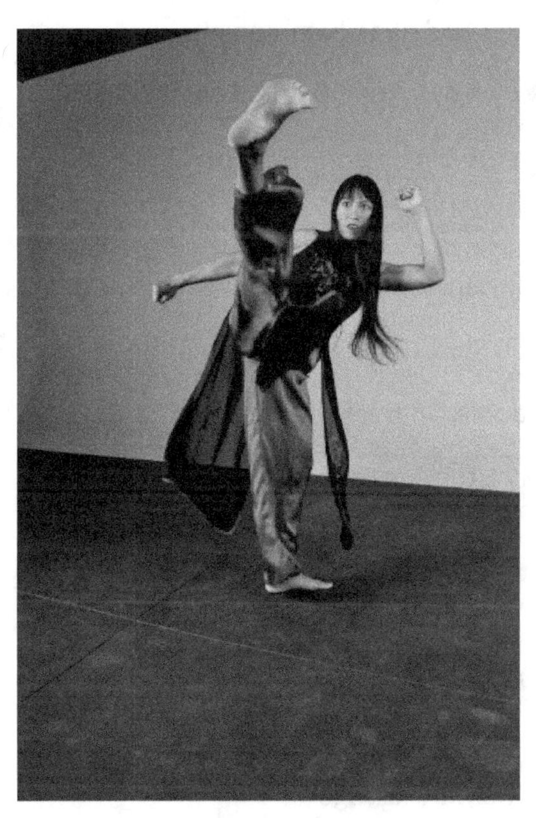

BOOKS AND DVDS FROM THE AUTHOR

The Mind of a Champion eBook

R.A.M.A. System Student Handbook

Create Your Best in 5 Steps

A Tender Heart Poetry Book

Shibashi Qigong Fountain of Wellness

Iron Shirt Qigong Transformation of Lifeforce

Doodle On from the Heart

My Little Poetry Book

DVDs

Dynamic Kicking

Dynamic Stretching

Dynamic Massage

A Girl from Ipanema Bonus Self-Defense

Shibashi Qigong Class

www.ingramcontent.com/pod-product-compliance
Lightning Source LLC
Chambersburg PA
CBHW051845250726
48659CB00006B/2027